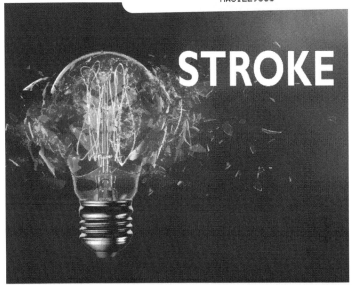

# STROKE

## Activities for the Family Caregiver
### *HOW TO ENGAGE, HOW TO LIVE*

*Endorsed by*

## National Council of
## Certified Dementia Practitioners

Scott Silknitter, Suzanne John
and Alisa Tagg

Disclaimer

This book is for informational purposes only and is not intended as medical advice, diagnosis, or treatment. Always seek advice from a qualified physician about medical concerns, and do not disregard medical advice because of something you may read within this book. This book does not replace the need for diagnostic evaluation, ongoing physician care, and professional assessment of treatments. Every effort has been made to make this book as complete and helpful as possible. It is important, however, for this book to be used as a resource and idea-generating guide and not as an ultimate source for plan of care.

ISBN 978-1-943285-23-5

Published by
R.O.S. Therapy Systems, L.L.C.
Greensboro, NC
888-352-9788
www.ROSTherapySystems.com

# Table of Contents

**Family Members and Caregivers
that have read this book:**

_____

_____

_____

_____

_____

_____

_____

_____

_____

_____

_____

_____

# Chapter 1

# Stroke Overview

In the simplest of terms, a stroke is defined as damage to the brain from an interruption of the blood supply. The medical terminology for a stroke is a cerebrovascular accident (CVA). It's critical to diagnose a stroke in progress because the treatment for stroke depends on the type of stroke, and, in some cases, the location of the injury to the brain. The American Stroke Association teaches the F.A.S.T. method—**F**ace drooping, **A**rm weakness, **S**peech difficulty, **T**ime to call 911.

Common complications after a stroke could be swelling of the brain, pneumonia, loss of bladder control, seizures, depression, pressure ulcers of the skin, contracted limbs, pain in the shoulder, and blood clotting.

An adaptation from the American Stroke Association, which gives a good overview of the stroke-related changes your loved one may experience, is below. You must be aware of these in order to adjust the assistance given and activities planned for your loved one.

## Common General Effects

- Weakness on one side of the body (Hemiparesis)
- Paralysis on one side of the body (Hemiplegia)
- Difficulty speaking or slurred speech (Dysarthria)
- Trouble swallowing (Dysphagia)
- Fatigue
- Loss of emotional control and changes in mood
- Cognitive changes (problems with memory, judgment, problem solving, or a combination of these)
- Behavior changes (personality changes, improper language, or actions)

- Decreased field of vision (inability to see peripheral vision) and trouble with visual impairment

Here is an example of how a stroke-related speech impairment can affect your loved one:

In response to any questions asked of her, Eloise is only able to state, "You can see what's coming." When asked if she would like to eat, Eloise responds the same. Depending on her tone and how she uses the phrase, it becomes easier to determine what she is wanting. While at an entertainment program, you notice that Eloise is singing along word-for-word with the entertainer. You engage in conversation with her and notice how excited she is to be singing along. Eloise is determined to speak using more words but easily becomes frustrated trying to use them. The caregiver discovers an easier way to help Eloise communicate for herself. They work together using scripted words to simple tunes. Eloise learns how to communicate through song.

A whole new world opens for her since she is able to sing her words rather than trying to speak. Music becomes the inspiration Eloise has been looking for.

The general effects of a stroke that can affect your loved one are determined by which side of the brain was damaged.

## Common Changes with Left-Brain Injury

- Paralysis or weakness on the right side of the body
- Aphasia (difficulty getting your words out or understanding what is being said)
- Behavior that may be more reserved and cautious than before

Here is an example of how Right-Side Paralysis can affect someone and how a properly trained caregiver can help.

Before her stroke, your mother, Lulu, enjoyed daily walks around her block. Since her stroke,

Lulu has been unable to take her walk, and she is becoming quite frustrated. You talk to Lulu about her frustration and discuss options that may allow her to have a regular walk again. The first idea is for you to push Lulu in her wheelchair around the block. Lulu states she would do this as a last resort. The caregiver then suggests using a walker, and a discussion is had with the Physical Therapist to determine Lulu's abilities. It is determined that Lulu can walk 100 feet using the walker before becoming tired and needing to rest. The caregiver discusses this with Lulu so she understands the situation. Together they decide that Lulu will walk the 100 feet using the walker and then ride in the wheelchair the rest of the way. Lulu is happy with the opportunity to get outside and enjoy this routine activity once again.

## Common Changes with Right-Brain Injury

- Paralysis or weakness on the left side of the body

- One-sided neglect, which is a lack of awareness of the left side of the body. It may also be a lack of awareness of what is going on to the survivor's left. For example, they may only eat from the right side of their plate, ignoring the left side.

- Behavior may be more impulsive and less cautious than before.

- It may be harder for the survivor to understand facial expressions and tone of voice. They also may have less expression in their own face and tone of voice when communicating.

Here is an example of how Left-Side Paralysis can affect your loved one because of right-side brain injury:

Since his stroke, Joe is unable to use his left arm. It is usually in a soft cast to help keep his hand from curling into a fist. Joe loves to play poker but has difficulty holding the cards anymore, and he becomes very frustrated when he has to lay them down in front of him on the table for others to see. The caregiver notices Joe's frustration and talks to him about using an adaptive device to hold playing cards. The adaptive device can easily keep the cards contained from others, and he is still able to work with them. Joe tries it out and is happy that he can still play cards without showing them to others.

## Common Emotional Effects of a Stroke

As with any major injury or issue, your loved one may experience emotional effects in addition to the physical damage. Some of the more common effects to be aware of with a stroke include:

- Depression
- Apathy and lack of motivation
- Frustration, anger, and sadness
- Pseudobulbar affect, also called reflex crying or emotional lability (emotions may change rabidly and sometimes not match the mood)

- Denial of the changes caused by the brain injury
- Frustration
- Anxiety
- Anger
- Changes in eating, sleeping, and thinking

As you and your loved one work through the physical and emotional issues associated with a stroke, you will also be thrust into the role of a caregiver. Patience is a virtue. As the primary caregiver, your patience will be tested, especially if you are tired or are in a stressful situation.

Your loved one may need more time to accomplish tasks, or they may not be able to answer questions the way they used to. The key is to be patient, and give your loved one the opportunity to be successful no matter the task. Make sure that all caregivers for your loved one understand that as well. There may be a point when caregivers have to step in and assist with tasks, but until that happens, give your loved one a chance to be successful and maintain self-confidence.

As the primary family caregiver—husband, wife, son, or daughter—your relationship and role with your loved one will change. You will become the cheerleader, motivator, protector, activity director, social coordinator, nurse, and maybe even mother or father to your loved one. You must prepare yourself for this role in the best way possible.

As a caregiver, there is no "job description" that explains what all caregivers do. Each caregiver's responsibilities vary according to the unique needs of the stroke survivor. Role changes and new skills may need to be learned. Common responsibilities of caregiving include:

- Providing physical help with personal care and transportation

- Managing financial, legal, and business affairs

- Monitoring behavior to ensure safety

- Managing housework and making meals

- Coordinating health care and monitoring or giving medications

- Helping the survivor maintain learned rehab skills and working to improve them

- Providing emotional support for the stroke survivor and family members

- Encouraging the stroke survivor to continue working toward recovery and to be as independent as possible

As the primary family caregiver, you need to know and understand the various symptoms of a stroke as previously stated so that you can adjust schedules, levels of participation, and the time it takes to participate accordingly. You will also need to educate family, friends, and other caregivers about what your loved one may be experiencing and why.

With activity and activities based on ***personal preference and ability***, people who have suffered from a stroke can still live a full life. One key to that is to engage in active activities, such as exercise, based on abilities. Exercise, including walking, working out on machines at your local gym, taking low-impact floor or water exercise classes, or doing yoga, can help reduce the risk of a stroke. It is also important to engage in mindful, creative, and social activities, such as playing cards, working crossword puzzles, playing checkers, talking with friends, painting, listening to music, or playing trivia games to keep the mind and parts of the body active. Use it or lose it, as the saying goes.

## Living at Home After a Stroke

Most stroke survivors are able to return home and resume many of the activities they did before the stroke.

Going home poses few problems for people who have had a minor stroke and have few lingering effects. For those whose strokes were more severe, going home depends on these factors:

- Ability to care for yourself. Rehabilitation should be focused on daily activities.

- Ability to follow medical advice. It is important to take medication as prescribed and follow medical advice.

- A caregiver—You. Someone who is willing and able to help when needed is essential.

- Ability to move around and communicate. If stroke survivors aren't independent in these areas, they may be at risk in an emergency, or they may feel isolated.

Planning, patience, effective communication, and the ability to adapt are all easier said than done if you are in the heat of the moment where everything that could happen, does happen. Please remember that your loved one did not choose to be here. If they could choose not to have suffered a stroke they would not have had it. You must use all of the resources available to you, such as this book, to be ready when something unexpected and/or unplanned does happen. Accept help when it is offered, and take time to take care of yourself whenever the opportunity arises. As much as it may feel like it at certain times, you are not alone in this fight.

# Chapter 2

# Activities, Their Benefits, and the Family

"Activities" refers to any endeavor, other than routine "Activities of Daily Living" (ADLs). A conversation, playing a game, working a puzzle, or taking a walk are all great examples of activities. For someone who has suffered a stroke, there may be challenges in participating in various activities. Because of that, activities should be planned to enhance your loved one's sense of well-being, and to promote or enhance their physical, cognitive, and emotional health.

In the institutional settings, activities are provided to every resident on a daily basis based on an individual's preferences. Activities has grown into a profession where Certified Activity Professionals and their staff plan and execute activity programs for residents and seniors in their care.

This book was written for the millions of families and informal caregivers who care for their loved ones who suffered from a stroke. Recognizing the growth in the numbers of those aging in place due to financial need or desire to just be at home, the R.O.S. Engagement Program and this book are based on the principles and approaches used by professionals in a skilled setting. This was done for two reasons.

1. Provide family caregivers the knowledge and tools to allow them to engage their loved one so that both can enjoy the benefits of activities.

2. Offer a starting point that will provide continuity of approach regarding care, communication, and information-gathering to minimize changes and acclimation time if your loved one does have to move from home to an institutional setting.

If you choose to use the services of a home care agency while caring for your loved one at home, please ask if they have a Home Care Certified professional on staff, and make sure that the caregiver you choose has received basic training on Activities and how to engage your loved one. This will assist with continuity of approach, communication, and planning that will benefit both you and your loved one.

Our goal is to help you deliver meaningful programs of interest to your loved one that focus on physical, social, spiritual, cognitive, and recreational activities. Everyone involved in caring for your loved one should be "on the same page" to minimize changes and challenges that your loved one will face. Therapeutic programs can also promote self-reliance and provide opportunities for creativity, self-expression, self-satisfaction, fun, and self-fulfillment. Some programs can specifically address managing stress, strengthening interpersonal skills, opportunities to learn new skills, or enhance skills your loved one already possesses.

# The Benefits of Activities with a Standard Approach

The benefits of being active and being engaged in activities are far-reaching for both you and your loved one. An Activities plan should be developed based on your loved one's personal preferences and abilities. Benefits include:

## Mental Benefits

Use is or lose it. Keeping your loved one's mind active is critical to helping them maintain their abilities and remain as sharp as possible.

## Social Benefits

Activities offer the opportunity for increased social interaction between family members, friends, caregivers, and the one being cared for. Activities create positive experiences and memories for everyone.

## Sleep Benefits

As part of a daily routine, activities can improve sleeping at night. If a loved one is inactive all day, it is likely they will nap periodically. Napping can interrupt good sleep patterns at night.

## Self-Esteem Benefits

Activities offered at the right skill level provide your loved one with an opportunity for success. Success during activities improves how your loved one feels about themselves.

## Anti-Depression and Anti-Anxiety Benefits

Engaging in activities can reduce symptoms of depression and anxiety. Research has shown a reduction in depression and anxiety through the provision of person-appropriate activities.

## Behavioral Benefits

Activities can reduce challenging behaviors when the activity conducted is interesting to your loved one. Offer activities at a skill level that allow your loved one to enjoy the activity.

## Caregiver Benefits

Activities result in less stress for the caregiver. When your loved one is participating in activities, there will be less of a need to respond to behavioral issues. This will allow for more opportunities to engage positively with one another.

Activities that your loved one with a stroke once enjoyed may still be accomplished; they just may be done a little differently.

Patience is vital. Adjustments must be made in preparation and execution to accommodate your loved one's remaining strengths and abilities.

## Activities, the Family, and Friends

Not all family members may understand or accept your loved one's situation following a stroke. This can create conflict. If it helps to avoid a conflict or stress, please have the family members read this book prior to a visit so they can begin to understand the monumental task that you face as a caregiver. Friends may also have a difficult time accepting the symptoms of a stroke. Use visits and interactions as teaching moments and to let the visitors know how much their visits mean to you and your loved one.

It can take a while to learn new roles and responsibilities. It is critical, however, to have as many family members and friends involved in your loved one's life as possible. Not just to show your loved one they are cared for, but also to give you, the primary family caregiver, the occasional and much-needed break.

The importance of understanding your family dynamics and the importance of each role an individual plays in the family will lead to better understanding and comprehension for the future.

Whether they come for an occasional visit or visit regularly every week, each family member can play an important role in your loved one's life. Family members can help with caregiving, preparing the home to ensure safety and quality of life, and successfully engaging with the loved one you care for.

## The Four Pillars of Activities

The R.O.S. Engagement Program focuses on the Four Pillars of Activities. These are areas that all caregivers for your loved one should be familiar with to provide continuity of care and give your loved one the greatest opportunity for success to engage and improve the quality of life for everyone.

### First Pillar of Activities: Know your Loved One—Information Gathering and Assessment

Have a Personal History Form completed. Know them—who they are, who they were, and what their functional abilities are today. Make sure all caregivers know this as well.

## Second Pillar of Activities: Communicating and Motivating for Success

Communication is key. Each caregiver must know how to effectively communicate with your loved one and be consistent with techniques.

## Third Pillar of Activities: Customary Routines and Preferences

As best as possible, maintain a routine and daily plan based on your loved one's needs and preferences.

## Fourth Pillar of Activities: Planning and Executing Activities

Based on all of the information you have gathered about your loved one, you have the opportunity to offer engaging activities that are appropriate and meet your loved one's personal preferences.

# Chapter 3

# First Pillar of Activities: Know Your Loved One— Information Gathering and Assessment

Knowing your loved one's individual needs, interests, functional abilities, and capacities will assist you in knowing how to plan and engage in meaningful and quality leisure activities. This is the First Pillar of Activities and will help in designing activities that your loved one can enjoy.

As the primary caregiver, you may already know most of the answers, but this is a good and necessary exercise for you, other family members, and other caregivers to execute. The following are items about your loved one that you are most likely able to provide yourself:

## Basic Information

Name, preferred name to be called, age, and date of birth

## Background Information

Place of birth, cultural/ethnic background, marital status, children (how many, and their names), religion/church, military service/employment, education level, and primary language spoken

## Medical and Dietary/Nutritional Information

Any formal diagnosis, allergies, and food regimen/diets

## Habits

Drinking/alcohol, smoking, exercise, and other things that are a daily habit

## Physical Status

Abilities/limitations, visual aids, hearing deficits, speech, communication, hand dominance, and mobility/gait

## Mental Status

Alertness; cognitive abilities/limitations; orientation to family, time, place, person, routine; ability to follow directions; preference for written or verbal instructions; ability to comprehend and follow one-step versus multi-step directions; safety awareness; safety concerns; etc.

## Social Status

One-on-one interaction; being visited; communication with others through written words, phone calls, or other means, such as email or online social networking services

## Emotional Status

Level of contentment, outgoing/withdrawn, extroverted/introverted, dependent/independent, easily frustrated, easygoing

## Leisure Status

Past, present, and possible future interests; solitary versus social activities; physical versus passive activities

## Vision Status

Any impairment they may have

# Informal Assessments

Informal assessments are done through interviews, observation, and information gathered through other means.

## Interviews

Interviews are conducted with your loved one, or with family members, friends, or significant others.

## Observations

An observation is what you and others have seen or heard concerning your loved one, e.g., how they interact with others, their behavior, and their responses to questions or statements made by others. This includes body language and expressions. You have probably seen these interactions a thousand times and made a mental note whenever something stuck out. Now, you must write them down for your future use and for others.

## Information Gathered Through Other Means

Make a request of family members or friends to help complete the Personal History Form at the back of this book. You also may download a copy of the Personal History Form at www.StartSomeJoy.org.

The interview process is particularly important for someone who has suffered from a stroke as they may become socially isolated. They may become easily embarrassed by their lack of motor control, which causes them to drop things, or they may grow tired of trying to explain things verbally when nonverbal expression is hindered by facial rigidity.

Help your loved one and others break through these barriers by gathering as much information as possible and sharing it with all caregivers—family, informal, and formal.

Your ability to identify past preferences is vital to the planning and execution of an activity, which we will cover in this book. Details matter. Let's look at someone who enjoys music.

During their assessments, three people might all say they like "music," yet they might not actually have the same activity in mind or enjoy the same activity.

- Person 1—Enjoys composing music and playing the piano.

- Person 2—Enjoys classical music and uses it to relax.

- Person 3—Enjoys fast-paced music and would listen to music when working out.

As you can see from these examples, details matter. Gather as much information as you can for yourself and all family members and caregivers who may help with your loved one.

The Personal History Form is a starting point to gather as much information as possible.

## Functional Levels

When reviewing person-appropriate abilities, in addition to the information from the American Stroke Association mentioned in Chapter 1, we must look at your loved one's functional levels. This will allow you to plan activities that your loved one can accomplish. There are many functional scales available, but for our purpose, we will use the five levels as follow.

### Level 1: Modified Independence

Your loved one is basically independent, using adaptive equipment or compensatory strategies. Social skills are adequate to make needs known and fit within the social norms. He or she initiates, plans, and even follows through with small projects/activities.

Those in this category have good social skills and are able to communicate. They are alert and oriented to person, place, and time, and they have a functional attention span for a concert or movie. They can initiate, plan, and even follow through with small projects/activities.

They also have problems with the big picture, responsibilities in family, follow through, attention to detail, and scheduling. They do not always think of the impact on others. They are ambulatory with or without a device. They may have lowered frustration tolerance and express frustration more readily.

## Level 2: Supervision

Your loved one at this level still has pretty good physical skills, ambulates with or without a device, and may drive. No physical assistance is needed, just verbal support— possibly as reminders to do exercise or use a cane or walker.

Those at this level can be more egocentric, less aware of others. Decreased social skills exist, such that those at Level 2 will yell at others who are slow or in the way. They need prompts to adjust tone or content of communication. They can participate in an activity with structure; set up and/or reminders; and prompting with sequencing, emotional regulation, and problem solving. They are somewhat rigid in ways and thinking.

**Level 3: Minimal Assistance**

At this level, your loved one may need both cognitive and physical assistance to complete tasks and participate in activities, but only about 25 percent of the time or with assistance for 25 percent of the task's effort. Support will need to be closer at hand in order to provide the assistance when needed. Memory and attention may be decreased, such that more routine prompting is needed in a 30 to 60 minute task; reminders are needed to finish or even stay on task. Support may be needed to give directions, such as to the bathroom in the movie theater or restaurant. Support might be needed in the form of a prompt to use a schedule and calendar. Physical and sensory deficits may require mild hands-on support, for instance holding hands or escorting when walking on uneven terrain or cues for walking across a street. You might notice endurance and fatigue levels are lower. The ability to make needs known may be affected by speech deficits or cognitive deficits. Your loved one has fewer social skills. His or her verbal skills are even more impaired than they were at Level 2. He or she is also easily distracted. Your loved one may have some visual/spatial perception and balance concerns, and needs maximum assistance with care.

## Level 4: Moderate–Maximum Assistance

At this level, someone is supporting your loved one in anywhere from 25–75 percent of a given task either cognitively, physically, or both. (The challenge may be physical or cognitive, but without the significant help from a caregiver, your loved one is unable to do the activity alone.)

Direct and more frequent prompts are needed for planning, problem solving, memory, and task attention. Initiation, safety awareness, and impulsivity can be a problem—requiring more supervision in the form of planning, encouragement, and safe execution of tasks. Physical and sensory deficits may be more severe, requiring assistance with self-care tasks as well as leisure activities. Increased physical assistance may be noted with the use of wheelchairs. Your loved one has a low energy level, few nonverbal communication skills, and rarely initiates contact with others; however, this person may respond if given time and cues.

## Level 5: Total Assistance

At this level, the physical and sensory deficits are more severe and limit the functional level. If the individual requires total care or is needing support for more than 75 percent of the given task, he or she is considered to be at the "total assistance" level of care. While this is most easily demonstrated by physical disabilities, if your loved one is mobile but has balance problems or tremors, for instance, and cognitive deficits that require constant supervision, constant prompting to stay on task and/or to be safe, and hand-over-hand assistance to engage, this person would be considered at Level 5, total assistance.

# Chapter 4

# Second Pillar of Activities: Communicating and Motivating for Success

Communicating and motivating for success is the Second Pillar for engaging in an activity with your loved one. The key to effective communication is the ability to listen attentively. This requires all caregivers to use communication techniques that provide an open, nonthreatening environment for your loved one. Listening behavior can either enhance and encourage communication or shut down communication altogether. You need to assess your listening style and be able to assess the listening styles of the other caregivers and family members working with your loved one.

# Verbal Communication

Communication is an interactive process where information is exchanged. The ability to respond appropriately, to give feedback on something that was communicated, is just as important as having good listening skills.

## Verbal Approaches

- Use exact, short, positive phrases. Repeat twice if necessary.

- Speak slowly.

- Allow time for your loved one to answer. Avoid finishing others' sentences.

- Give one instruction at a time. Provide only the number of steps your loved one can handle at a time.

- Use a warm, gentle tone of voice.

- There is no need to shout, unless your loved one also has a hearing impairment.

- If your loved one is unable to see you because of a visual impairment, be sure to use verbal cues to let them know you are engaged.

- Talk to your loved one like an adult.

- Only use words your loved one is familiar with.

## Verbal Communication Tips

- Make your presence known when entering a room by saying hello.

- Identify yourself. Do not assume the person knows or remembers who you are.

- If there are others present, address your loved one by name so there is no confusion as to whom you are speaking.

- Indicate the end of a conversation, and be sure your loved one knows when you leave so that they aren't left talking to an empty space.

- Speak directly to your loved one.

- Always answer questions, and be specific or descriptive in your responses.

- When giving directions, make the directions as clear as possible. Use "left" and "right" according to the way your loved one is facing.

- Provide a written summary of information/instructions as needed if memory is an issue.

- When speaking with other caregivers or family members about your loved one while they are present, make sure the conversation is respectful of your loved one, and be sure to include your loved one in the conversation to avoid it being "about" them.

- Avoid battles or direct confrontations. For example, avoid situations wherein you are telling someone to do something.

## Nonverbal Communication

Although it may seem that most communication happens verbally, research has shown that actually most communication occurs nonverbally. Nonverbal communication occurs through an individual's body language. Do not assume that nonverbal communication does not matter to someone who has visual impairment due to a stroke or some other factor just because you "think" it does not.

A loved ones who experienced a stroke may have developed aphasia.

### Effects of Aphasia
- Trouble speaking
- Trouble finding words
- Problems understanding what others say
- Problems with reading, writing, or math
- Inability to process long words and infrequently used words

People with aphasia are often frustrated and confused because they can't speak as well or understand things the way they did before their stroke. They may act differently because of changes in their brain. Imagine looking at the headlines of the morning newspaper and not being able to recognize the words. Or think about trying to say, "Put the car in the garage," and it comes out, "Put the train in the house," or "Widdle tee car ung sender plissen." Thousands of alert, intelligent men and women are suddenly plunged into a world of jumbled communication because of aphasia.

## Types of Aphasia

- Global Aphasia (both expressive and receptive)—People with this aphasia may be completely unable to speak, name objects, repeat phrases, or follow commands.

- Broca's Aphasia (expressive)—The person knows what they want to say,

but can't find the right words
(can't "get the words out").

- Wernicke's Aphasia (receptive)—A
person with this aphasia can seldom
understand what's being said or control
what they're saying.

- The challenge for caregivers is to provide
people with aphasia a means to express
what they know.

When someone has aphasia:

- It is important to make the distinction
between language and intelligence.

- Many people mistakenly think they are
not as smart as they used to be.

- Their problem is that they cannot
use language to communicate what
they know.

- They can think—they just can't say what
they think.

- They can remember familiar faces.

- They can get from place to place.

- They still have political opinions.

- They may still be able to participate in activities they once participated in.

The point is that aphasia does not affect intelligence. Stroke survivors remain mentally alert, even though their speech may be jumbled, fragmented, or impossible to understand. Nonverbal communication becomes more important. There are five key elements to consider:

**Facial Expressions**

Be aware of what your facial expressions are conveying to your loved one. Your mood will be mirrored.

**Eye Contact**

Ensure that you have made eye contact with your loved one and that their attention is focused on you and what you are saying.

## Gestures and Touch

Calmly use nonverbal signs, such as pointing, waving, and other hand gestures in combination with your words.

## Tone of Voice

The inflection in your voice helps your loved one relate to the words you are saying.

## Body Language

Be aware of the position of your hands and arms when talking to your loved one.

*Note: When communicating with your loved one, be mindful that their body language may not fully tell how they feel or what they are trying to express because of their stroke. Your body language, however, will be read by your loved one.

## Nonverbal Communication Tips

- Always approach your loved one from the front before speaking to them.

- Smile and extend your hand as to shake their hand. Use touch where welcomed.
- Do not touch unexpectedly; it might startle your loved one.
- Place yourself at eye level with the loved one with whom you are speaking.
- Use nonverbal gestures along with words.
- Give nonverbal praises, such as smiles and head nods.
- Be an active listener.
- Make sure that all caregivers give your loved one the opportunity and time to speak.

# Approaches to
# Successful Communication & Activities

### Be Calm

Always approach your loved one in a relaxed and calm demeanor. Remember, your mood will be mirrored by your loved one. Smiles are contagious.

## Be Flexible

There is no right or wrong way of completing a task. Offer praise and encouragement for the effort your loved one puts into a task. If you see your loved one becoming overwhelmed or frustrated, stop the task, and re-approach at another time.

## Be Nonresistive

Don't force tasks on your loved one. Adults do not want to be told, "No!" or told what to do. The power of suggestion goes a long way, and you get more with an ounce of sugar than you do a pound of vinegar.

## Be Guiding, but Not Controlling

Always use a soft, gentle approach, and remember your tone of voice. Your facial expressions must match the words you are saying.

## Barriers to Good Communication

Caregiver barriers and environmental barriers can negatively affect communication with your loved one.

### Caregiver Barriers to Communication

Make sure that you and everyone that comes in to assist with your loved one are on the same page and use the same verbal communication approaches. Some tips to eliminate caregiver barriers include:

- Slow down when speaking too quickly. Also, speak clearly.

- Use a calm tone of voice, and be aware of your hand movements.

- Never be demanding or commanding.

- Never argue with a person with impaired cognition. You will never win the argument.

- Do not offer long explanations when answering questions.

- Do not let your anger and frustration at various situations build and turn into hurtful words.

## Environmental Barriers to Communication

With so many things happening around us, we must make sure to remove, or adapt to, avoidable communication barriers around us. Here are some examples:

- Minimize noise from air conditioners and home appliances.
- Turn off the TV if it is on in the same room where you are trying to talk.
- Be aware of outside traffic noise.
- Check hearing aid batteries to ensure they are not whistling.
- Adjust the lighting in the room. If the lighting in a room negatively affects your loved one's vision, they may be more focused on trying to see rather than on communicating with you.

# Chapter 5

# Third Pillar of Activities:
## Customary Routines
## and Preferences

Customary routines and preferences is the Third Pillar in an activities program. Activities can occur all day every day. The question should not be, "When should I do activities?" It is not important to focus on when to do activities. The focus should be on making each and every interaction memorable and always respecting your loved one as an individual.

For the purpose of developing a daily plan of care, we will be discussing two areas: Daily Customary Routine and Activity Preferences. The goal is to gain from your loved one's perspective how important certain aspects of care/activity are of interest to them as an individual.

**Daily Customary Routine**

Your loved one has distinct lifestyle preferences and routines. They should be preserved to the greatest extent possible. All reasonable accommodation should be made to maintain their lifestyle preferences.

Not accommodating your loved one's lifestyle preferences and routine can contribute to depressed mood or increased behavior symptoms or potentially dangerous situations. When a person feels like their control has been removed and that their preferences are not respected as an individual, it can be demoralizing. The little things matter. Let us look at an example:

Since his stroke, Bill has become more impulsive, trying to get out of his chair to do something, and has had multiple falls. Bill's children are concerned that he could injure himself by falling.

Bill's primary caregiver, his daughter Susan, discusses this concern with Bill in order to come up with a resolution. Bill says that he is forgetful about the fact that he cannot walk anymore, but he still wants to be independent. Susan and Bill work together on a game plan to help him have his independence. The plan includes reminders for Susan to ask Bill if he needs to move or use the restroom.

As part of his daily routine, Bill enjoys watching TV after breakfast. Susan had noticed Bill getting up frequently while he was watching TV and she was cleaning up from breakfast. She realized one of the reasons that Bill had been trying to get up was to grab the remote control which had always been kept on a table across the room. Part of Susan's plan now included placing the remote control and other items Bill may need within his reach. The little things matter.

**Activity Preferences**

Activities are a way for individuals to establish meaning in their lives. The need for enjoyable activities does not change based on their age or health needs. The only thing that changes is the level of assistance they may need in order to engage in those pursuits.

A lack of opportunity to engage in meaningful and enjoyable activities can result in boredom, depression, and behavioral disturbances.

Individuals vary in the activities they prefer, reflecting unique personalities, past interest, perceived environmental constraints, religious and cultural background, and changing physical and mental abilities. We as family caregivers have a great opportunity to empower a loved one to see that they possess many great talents and abilities. By modifying or adapting an activity to allow them to engage at an independent level, you are restoring their self-esteem and self-worth.

Let's use an everyday exercise routine.

- Person 1—Enjoys going outside for a daily two-mile walk.

  After a stroke, Person 1 has one-side paralysis, and now he uses a quad cane to get around.

  Adaptation: Encourage him to take slower, shorter, supervised walks up and down the driveway. He can gradually increase his walks to the corner and back multiple times during the day rather than all at once.

- Person 2—Enjoys lifting heavy weights three times a week.

  After a stroke, Person 2 is no longer able to lift weights as she was used to. This has caused a lot of frustration in Person 2.

  Adaptation: Utilize soup cans or water bottles filled with dry beans for weights to provide exercises for the side that has full range of motion. On the affected side, utilize cut-up pool foam noodles for easier hold and encourage maximum participation.

- Person 3—Enjoys swimming on a daily basis.

  After a stroke, Person 3 is worried that with paralysis he will no longer be able to swim.

  Adaptation: Use the local pool for walking laps utilizing a kickboard for stability. Ensure a caregiver is in the water for support.

- Person 4—Enjoys doing yoga.

  A stroke left Person 4 with the inability to perform the yoga poses that she was used to doing.

  Adaptation: Introduce wheelchair yoga so she can practice on a seated level.

# Chapter 6

# Fourth Pillar of Activities: Planning and Executing Activities

Planning and executing activities is the Fourth Pillar in engaging a loved one in an activity. In order to do that, activities can be spontaneous, but generally must be planned and appropriate for your loved one in order to offer the greatest opportunity for success. Please note that schedules, routines, and plans should be followed. However, they may need to be adapted due to specific issues your loved one may be experiencing that day.

As you plan your loved one's activities as part of the customary routine, you need to consider how an activity fits within the following criteria:

- Person Appropriate—Desires and Preferences
- Person Appropriate—Abilities and Functional Levels

## Person Appropriate— Desires and Preferences

"Person appropriate" refers to the idea that each person has a personal identity and history. It means that the caregiver has to make sure that all caregivers understand the concept of a specific activity because the name of the activity can mean different things to different people.

Remember our music example:

- Person 1—Enjoys composing music and playing the piano.

- Person 2—Enjoys classical music and uses it to relax.

- Person 3—Enjoys fast-paced music and would listen to music when working out.

Remember, when planning activities, you need to ensure that the activity is person appropriate, based on the specific desires and preferences of your loved one.

## Person Appropriate— Abilities and Functional Levels

This concept is also based on the idea that each person has a personal identity and history, but it also takes into account the varying functional levels at which a person may be able to participate in an activity. The effects of age, declining health, recovery from a stroke, and other diseases on a person's physical and mental abilities, at some point may mean that while many activities can still be performed, some activities may be facilitated through certain modifications, e.g., by using adaptive equipment.

Based on your loved one's functional level and abilities, some activities may also be done as a group activity. This creates an opportunity for socialization, interaction, and conversation between you and your loved one.

# The Lesson Plan

In order to keep all caregivers up-to-date and informed as to your loved one's ability to participate in an activity after a stroke, we suggest using an activity Lesson Plan to document everything.

The Lesson Plan template at the end of this chapter is a guideline for an activity. It is an ever-changing document. It is meant to be written on to note the changes you made in the original plan so the family member or caregiver working with your loved one next can follow your modifications in the hopes of recreating a positive experience.

## Items in the Lesson Plan

### Date

Document the date the activity is used with your loved one.

### Activity Name

Give the activity a name that you or your loved one prefers.

## Objective of Activity

Our goal is to provide meaningful activities. People have a need to be productive, and they want to engage in something with a purpose. List the objectives of the activity.

## Materials

List suggested materials to be used with this activity.

## Prerequisite Skills

List the skills your loved one needs in order to participate in this activity.

## Room Lighting

List the lighting conditions that will allow your loved one to be successful in engaging with the activity.

## Activity Outline

List the step-by-step instructions to complete this activity.

## Evaluation

When you or a family member is conducting an activity with your loved one, documenting results and responses is critical to identifying ways to improve activity programs for your loved one. Items to document should include:

- Verbal cues, physical assistance, or modifications you required for this activity.
- How your loved one responded to this activity.
- Whether your loved one enjoyed this activity. What did they like or dislike about the activity?
- Whether the activity was successful at distracting or eliminating a negative behavior. Why and how was it successful?

A blank template is included on the next page to give you an example of what a Lesson Plan looks like.

**\*Note:** Make sure caregivers and family members are consistent with the type of verbal cues, physical assistance, or modifications that produce positive results.

## Lesson Plan Blank Example

| Date | Activity Name |
|------|---------------|

**Objective of Activity**

**Materials**

**Prerequisite Skills**

**Room Lighting**

**Activity Outline**

**Evaluation**

# Chapter 7

# Leisure Activity Categories, Tips, and Suggestions

## Activity Categories

Activities are generally broken down into three different categories: maintenance activities, supportive activities, and empowering activities.

### Maintenance Activities

Maintenance activities are traditional activities that help your loved one maintain physical, cognitive, social, spiritual, and emotional health. Examples include:

- Using manipulative games, such as those from R.O.S. Therapy Systems

- Craft and art activities

- Attending church services

- Working trivia and crossword puzzles like the R.O.S. *How Much Do You Know About* puzzle series on www.Amazon.com or www.TheROSStore.com
- Taking a walk

**Supportive Activities**

If your loved one has a lower tolerance for traditional activities, supportive activities provide a comfortable environment while providing stimulation or solace. Examples include:

- Listening to and singing music
- Hand massages
- Relaxation activities, such as aromatherapy, meditation, and bird-watching

**Empowering Activities**

Empowering activities help your loved one attain self-respect by offering opportunities for self-expression and exercising responsibility. Examples include:

- Cooking
- Making memory boxes
- Folding laundry

## General Activity Tips

### Travel Tips for Moving from Room to Room or Place to Place

- When escorting your loved one, ask them if they need assistance. If they do not request any assistance, walk side-by-side or a half step behind.

- If your loved one experiences complications from the stroke, please remember your communication techniques—be calm, be flexible, be guiding, but not controlling. There is no need to yell or startle your loved one while they are working through taking a step. If you are in public, yelling may draw unwanted attention to them, causing them to focus on potentially being embarrassed rather than on taking a step. Be patient.

- If your loved one does require some assistance, offer your arm for your loved one to hold onto or interlock with. Find the easiest and most comfortable way to walk together. Walk side-by-side or a half pace ahead while providing verbal cues about the environment.

- Announce when you are approaching doorways, stairs, and ramps.

- Avoid puddles, snowbanks, and other natural barriers.

- Avoid cracked tile, untacked throw rugs, and protruding floorboards.

## Writing and Coloring Activity Tips

- If your loved one has trouble holding a pen or pencil, wrap foam around the shaft of the pen to help your loved one's grip. You can try cutting a piece from a foam noodle used in a swimming pool to fit on the writing tool.

- Reduce glare and shadowing by positioning a chair and table so any natural light is behind them instead of coming at them from the front.

- To prevent shadows, place lamps on the opposite side of the hand being used. Locate the bottom edge of the lampshade just below eye level.

- Shiny paper can increase glare, so it's best to use matte paper when reading or writing.

- Use large-print crossword, word search, or word scramble puzzles. If you cannot find the R.O.S. *How Much Do You Know About* puzzle series or other large-print sources, most copiers have the ability to increase the size of the print.

- A dry-erase board or tablet may also be used to practice writing.

* **Note:** Know the type of seating where your loved one is the most comfortable when they are writing, and, if possible, move them to that seat.

* **Note:** If your loved one is seated in wheelchair, recliner, or bed, provide a flat surface that fits in their lap to place paper on.

## Reading Activity Tips

- Large-print books are available at most bookstores and libraries.

- Read to your loved one, or take turns reading to each other.

- Listen to audio tapes and books on CD borrowed from your local library, or from the free Talking Books program sponsored by the National Library Service.

- If your loved one prefers reading to listening, many new mobile devices, such as iPads, Kindles, and Nooks all have options to increase the font size and adjust the color contrast.

- Try the Book Strap from R.O.S. Therapy Systems to help keep a book and the page in place.

## Craft Activity Tips

- Make sure that supplies are easily accessible.

- Empower your loved one by choosing an area of the home where they can most comfortably participate.

    ○ If at a table and in a wheelchair, make sure the wheelchair can fit under the table.

    ○ If in a recliner, use an activity surface that fits comfortably in their lap, and choose an activity that does not have too many pieces that may be hard to keep track of.

- Craft Boxes and Materials
  - ○ Place craft activity supplies in boxes clearly labeled with a broad-tipped black marker.
  - ○ Group like items for activities together.
  - ○ Store materials in different shaped/sized containers for easier recognition.
  - ○ Choose identifying and organizational systems that work best for your loved one.

## Music Tips

Music has health benefits. Listening to music can help with common complications that occur among people after a stroke.

People who have aphasia are able to express themselves more freely through music. They communicate best through music.

People who listen to music for one hour a day for one week—whether they picked the tunes themselves or researchers provided them—felt more empowered, and reported less pain, depression, and disability than those who did not listen to music. Average pain ratings among people who listened to music fell by about 20 percent, whereas pain among nonlisteners actually increased.

Classical music is one of the best choices. Listening to slow-tempo classical music may ease pain. Music can be very powerful.

If classical music isn't your cup of tea, try jazz or new age genres. Here are a few suggestions of healing music:

- Beethoven for Relaxation
- Chopin for Relaxation
- Vivaldi for Relaxation
- Music for Sound Healing

If you don't have an iPod or radio handy, singing works as well.

**Game Playing Activity Tips**

Playing Cards:

- If needed, use adaptive equipment to place the playing cards in while your loved one is seated at a table.

- The Card Holder Board Insert from R.O.S. Therapy Systems allows your loved one to have the card holder in their lap, hands-free, while seated in a recliner or wheelchair.

Puzzles:

- Choose puzzles with larger pieces. These are easier for your loved one to manipulate.

- If your loved one becomes frustrated because puzzle pieces are sliding when being placed, try a magnetic puzzle and a metallic flat surface so the pieces stick when placed.

## Active Activity Suggestions

In addition to the tips for general activities, please review the following suggestions for active activities. As you build these activities into your loved one's life, please make sure to schedule opportunities for rest after or between activities.

Active activities can be broken into four areas that all can help improve the quality of life for your loved one.

### Aerobic Activities

During aerobic activities, the body's large muscles move in a rhythmic manner for a sustained period of time. Aerobic activities help to maintain or improve cardiovascular health.

### Strengthening Activities

Strengthening activities improve overall muscle strength, walking speed, posture, and overall physical fitness.

## Flexibility Activities

Flexibility or stretching exercises improve mobility, increase range of motion, reduce stiffness, and can help reduce the risk of injury.

## Balance Activities

Balance activities improve posture and stability.

**\*Note**: Depending on the activity or exercise, you, a family member, or a trained professional should always be there to supervise and assist your loved one as needed.

# Aerobic Activities

Objectives of aerobic activities include improving physical fitness and having positive effects on slowness, stiffness, and mood.

Examples of aerobic activities for your loved one:

- Walking
    - with you, a family member, or your dog
    - on a treadmill
    - around the shopping mall
- Swimming or water aerobics
    - at your gym or YMCA
- Dancing
    - at home with you, a family member, or a friend
    - at a local dance hall, club, or ballet center
- Chair aerobics
    - in your living room following along with a video
    - at your local gym or YMCA

## Strengthening Activities

The objective of improving muscle strength is to facilitate everyday activities, such as getting up from a chair, moving from room to room in the home, and making any task easier to manage.

Examples of strengthening activities for your loved one:

- Weights/resistance
  - ○ free weight activities/exercises
  - ○ elastic bands activities/exercises
  - ○ body weight activities/exercises
- Yard work or gardening

What strengthening activities will your loved one enjoy, and where will they be done?

## Flexibility Activities

Objectives of stretching and flexibility activities include improving range of motion, which can affect posture and walking ability, reducing the risk of injury, and making every-day activities easier.

Examples of flexibility activities for your loved one:

- Gentle stretching
  - ○ In your living room following along with a video

- Yoga, including chair yoga
- Bilateral arm training with rhythmic auditory cueing (BATRAC)
- Treadmill-supported walking
- Strengthening or resistance training

## Balance Activities

Balance activities can improve posture and stability. Preserving your loved one's ability to maintain their balance can help to reduce the likelihood of falling, potentially calm your loved one's fears of falling, and help them generally in performing daily tasks.

Examples of balance activities for your loved one:

- Yoga, including chair yoga
- At-home balance exercises using
  - A Wii
  - A balance ball or balance pillow

What balance activities will your loved one enjoy, and where will they be done?

75

# Chapter 8

# Activities of Daily Living Tips and Suggestions

Unlike the leisure activities discussed, the activities of daily living covered in this book are activities that are a necessary part of everyday life. The following pages contain tips and suggestions for you to use with your loved one. These tips are particularly helpful for those functioning at a level that requires moderate to total assistance.

## Energy Conservation and Rest

The body requires tremendous energy to heal itself. Energy conservation and rest can be important based on your loved one's unique situation. You, as the caregiver, have to decide that. As the day is scheduled, make sure to plan periods of rest between activities.

The simplification of daily tasks will conserve energy for your loved one. If your loved one uses less energy on one task, it can help them have more energy for other activities throughout the day. Your loved one will expend different levels of energy with different activities (bathing, dressing, toileting, etc.). Evaluate your loved one's performance of an activity and decide if it is performed as efficiently as possible. Never underestimate the energy needed for activities requiring a lot of thought (cognition)—in addition to the obvious physical effort required for an activity. Even when your loved one is experiencing post-stroke physical and/or cognitive impairments, you always want to encourage your loved one to be as independent as safely possible.

All activities of the day should be planned out to the greatest extent possible—this includes personal care routines, leisure activities, chores, and exercise. They should be spaced throughout the day, with the activities that require the most energy being accomplished at the time of day your loved one feels the best.

Do not schedule too many things to do in one day, and be prepared to cancel some plans if your loved one is not feeling well or up to it. It is better to do fewer things over a few days than try to do them all in one day and create exhaustion and possible physical discomfort for days because of poor pacing.

Discuss with your loved one, ahead of time, your level of assistance with certain activities on days with higher activities or when an additional activity is being incurred. For example, Grandma usually takes 45 minutes to dress, toilet, and brush her teeth in the morning, and she has a 30-minute nap two hours after that activity. Today, you are taking her to a doctor appointment at 1:00 p.m. If you assist with the dressing portion of her morning activity, she can conserve and utilize that energy for the doctor's appointment. While efficient planning is your greatest asset, the ability to adjust and accommodate other circumstances is vital. Remember to openly communicate the day's events and encourage independence in activities as safety permits.

If your loved one becomes tired during an activity, allow for pause and rest. If your loved one turns a rest period into a nap, be careful not to let the nap go too long during the day, as sleep may become elusive at night. Keeping awake and sleep patterns is important, as are activities.

## Bathing

Bathing can be a relaxing, enjoyable experience—or a time of confrontation and anger. If your loved one needs assistance with bathing, use a calm approach. Your loved one's "usual" routine is very important.

### Safety and Preparation

- Water temperature should range from 110– 115 degrees Fahrenheit maximum to prevent burning or skin injury. Use your elbow to check the water temperature—hands are not consistent indicators of temperatures.

- Hot water can cause fatigue.

- The floor of the tub needs to be slip resistant. Use a rubber mat that doesn't slide, or use permanent nonslip decals.

- Place a nonskid rug on the floor outside the tub to prevent slipping.

- Install grab bars. Always make sure the grab bars are properly and securely installed into the wall studs.

- Utilize a bath/shower chair if necessary.

## Bathing—Know Your Loved One

- Is your loved one accustomed to a bath or shower?

- Does your loved one need assistance to get into the bath or shower?

- Can your loved one soap their body or wash their hair alone?

- Can your loved one independently dry with a towel? A simple trick is to sew straps onto the towel to make the towel easier to hold.

- If help is needed, who is your loved one the most comfortable with when bathing?

- It can be awkward waiting and watching someone perform such a personal task. As the caregiver, you can provide supervision, but be involved in another activity within the space. For instance, getting towels out while your loved one is undressing is an effective use of time. Washing your loved one's lower body while they wash their upper body can deflect this discomfort. This also creates a sense of support versus a feeling of total dependence.

**Bathing—Communicating and Motivating**

If you have to help a loved one bathe:

- Allow your loved one to do what is safely within their control.

- Stay friendly and respectful. Be "gently guiding".

- Try to avoid arguments by offering a combination of visual cues, step-by-step setup, and short verbal cues.

**Bathing—Customary Routines and Preferences**

- What time of day does your loved one normally bathe?

- How often did your loved one bathe prior to the stroke?

- What is the process that works for you and your loved one when it is time to bathe? Make sure all caregivers know each detail of the process.

For example, is the water turned on and running prior to your loved one entering the tub? Is a towel placed on a shower chair that your loved one may use so that the chill on his or her bottom is removed when sitting?

- Whatever the process, take it one step at a time, following the person's normal bathing routine. For example, the loved one may prefer that you wash their hair first and then their body. If sitting in the tub, they may like to soak for 10 minutes before washing.

- When assisting your loved one, have a towel ready to put over their shoulders or on their lap to minimize feelings of exposure. Maintain privacy—close blinds, curtains, and doors. Avoid drafts.

- Be sure to have your loved one's favorite personal care products for familiar smell and feeling. Making a bath/shower caddy of their favorite products is a good idea.

### Bathing—Planning and Executing

- Have all care items and tools ready prior to starting the bath process.

  ○ A shower chair if necessary

  ○ A handheld hose for showering and bathing

  ○ A long-handled sponge or scrubbing brush if self-scrubbing is desired

  ○ Sponges with soap inside or a soft soap applicator instead of bar soap (bar soap can easily slip out of your loved one's hand)

- Have a towel and clothing prepared for when the bath is finished.

- A second towel can be placed on the back of a chair to allow your loved one to dry his or her back by rubbing on the towel or you might use a terry cloth robe instead of a towel for drying.

- Always use bath time to observe and assess your loved one's skin health. Document any concerns or changes that you might notice, and use this as a communication tool with other caregivers.

## Other Bathroom & Grooming Activities

Encourage your loved one to maintain personal grooming habits. Your loved one may need physical or cognitive assistance or both. If your loved one has participated in occupational therapy, utilize the adaptive and compensatory strategies and tips from rehabilitation for optimum independence. For example, you may need to set up the space so that bathing items are easy to reach, adjust shower seating, or use a handheld shower, a checklist for the steps of the task, or teamwork for the hardest parts of the task.

It can sometimes be easier to "do things" for your loved one to save time and mess. In the long run, this serves to make your loved one more dependent. Encouraging independence for as long as possible is a key goal and is essential to your loved one's overall health.

- Allow plenty of time for routines. If having your loved one do everything independently takes more time than available, select two to four tasks that are most important. Keep the big picture in mind. Your loved one may value being outdoors, volunteering, or exercising more. If time is a factor, save time in personal care routines, and spend time on the activities that bring your loved one the most satisfaction. Communicate and reach agreements on how you can assist. This allows your loved one to feel in "control" and fosters feelings of independence.

- Having someone brush your loved one's teeth is not always a comfortable feeling. Always allow him or her to do what is safely possible. Adaptive grips might help for holding onto the toothbrush. Electric brushes can compensate for fine motor deficits and often include a timer indicating how long to brush.

- Helping your loved one maintain oral hygiene is very important for those who can no longer do it themselves or do it thoroughly. Poor hygiene can lead to additional health problems including gum disease, mouth sores, and infections.

Encourage your loved one to keep up with personal grooming, such as shaving, makeup application, and hair care. Provide physical assistance as needed. Large grip items may help with fine motor challenges.

- Use an electric razor for safety.

- Give positive feedback, and avoid pointing out small mistakes. Be gently guiding in your approach.

- If your loved one had been accustomed to wearing makeup, there is no reason for this to stop. If your loved one shows interest or a desire to wear makeup, encourage the familiar routine and offer assistance to apply it if needed. Explore built-up grips for brushes and combs. Consider teaching them to stabilize the elbow on the counter or sink to provide more control of the hand.

## Hair

- Try to maintain the hairstyle and hair care routine to which your loved one is familiar. However, if independence is more important, consider a style that allows this independence.

## Toileting or Using the Bathroom

- Learn your loved one's individual toileting habits and routines. This might not be something you needed knowledge of before the stroke, but it is necessary now to accommodate your changing role in your loved one's care.

- The best approach is to offer the toilet routinely on rising, both in the morning and upon awakening from a nap. Also, offer the toilet at least 30 to 40 minutes after meals and at bedtime at minimum. You will readily learn your loved one's habits, notice when changes occur, and notice when outside factors might influence changes. It is recommended to keep a record or journal to communicate this routine with other caregivers.

- If your loved one suffers with communication difficulties due to the stroke, watch for nonverbal clues, such as agitation, pulling at the clothes, crying, or restlessness. This may indicate a need to use the bathroom.

- When needed, help with clothing, and be positive and pleasant while assisting.

- Provide verbal cues and instructions as needed. Be guiding, but not controlling.

- If your loved one has fine motor deficits or hemiplegia, clothing with minimal fasteners, elastic-waist pants, or stretch pants can be more easily pulled up/down and help make toileting less difficult.

- Be sure to provide other caregivers/ providers information regarding the toileting schedule of your loved one when they are outside the home setting.

- Know the public toilet access prior to going somewhere. Not all public bathrooms are user friendly, despite being "accessible." This will help reduce any possible anxiety your loved one may have in regards to toileting when on an outing.

## Clothing

### Clothing—Know Your Loved One

- Your loved one may return to the same style of clothes worn before the stroke.

- If personal care is a challenge, clothes need to be comfortable and easy to remove, especially for toileting.

- Choose clothes that are loose fitting and have elastic waistbands. Items with larger buttons are easier to manipulate.

- If possible, choose clothing that opens in the front, not the back. This prevents your loved one from having to reach behind the body and encourages independence when dressing.

- When the stroke has caused deficits with your loved one's motor skills, look for clothing with large, flat buttons, Velcro closures, zippers, or elastic waistbands when purchasing new items of clothing.

- To assist your loved one with zipping pants or a jacket, attach a zipper pull or leather loop on the end of the zipper.

- If bending and tying shoes is problematic, consider slip-on shoes. Non-tie shoes are very popular now. There are also elastic type shoestrings that allow previously tied shoes to become slip-ons.

## Clothing—Routines and Preferences

- If your loved one has trouble paying attention and making choices, you may have to limit the clothing choices you offer, and leave only two outfit options in the room at a time.

- If your loved one wants to wear the same thing every day, and if you can afford it, buy three or four sets of the same clothing.

## Clothing—Planning and Executing

- Clothes should be laid out according to what goes on first. This should be determined by your loved one's preferred routine.

- Avoid clothes that are most difficult for your loved one, such as panty hose, knee-high nylons, tight socks, or high heels.

- Make sure that items are not inside out and that buttons, zips, and fasteners are all undone before handing the clothes to your loved one.

- Be sure clothing is neat and clean. Appearance influences one's dignity and self-esteem.

## Dressing

### Dressing—Know Your Loved One

Your loved one may just need verbal cues and instructions on dressing. Please remember to allow independent dressing as much as possible to foster an ongoing sense of dignity and independence. Be gently guiding. As the primary caregiver, you will need to assess when your loved one's abilities change and instruct all caregivers to assist accordingly.

## Dressing—Communicating and Motivating

- When providing instruction to your loved one, use short simple sentences.

- If your loved one is confused, give instructions in very short steps, such as, "Now put your arm through the sleeve." It is helpful to use actions to demonstrate these instructions.

- Remember to offer the toilet before getting dressed.

- Avoid "hovering" while your loved one is dressing. You need to be available as needed during the process, but you can do another task, like make the bed or straighten up, so your loved one does not feel so slow or incompetent, or that you are waiting on them.

## Dressing—Routines and Preferences

- Does your loved one get dressed first thing in the morning—before breakfast or after breakfast?

94

- Does your loved one change into pajamas right before bed or after dinner?

- Try to maintain your loved one's preferred routine for as long as possible.

- Little things matter. For example, your loved one may like to put on all underwear before putting on anything else.

## Dressing—Planning and Executing

- If there are others living in the house, remember to provide privacy. Close blinds or curtains, close the door, and put a do not disturb "dressing" sign out to ensure privacy.

- If your loved one suffers from one-sided weakness (hemiplegia) or left neglect as a stroke complication, the rule for dressing is to dress the weak side first. When removing clothes it is recommended that you undress the strong (unaffected) side first.

- If mistakes are made—for example, by putting something on the wrong way—be tactful, or find a way for both of you to laugh about it.

**\*Note:** Wearing several layers of thin clothing rather than one thick layer can be helpful. With layers, your loved one will be able to remove a layer if too warm. Remember that your loved one may not be able to tell you if he or she gets too hot or cold, so keep an eye out for signs of discomfort.

## Eating

### Eating—Know Your Loved One

- Keep long-standing personal preferences in mind when preparing food. However, be aware that your loved one may suddenly develop new food preferences or reject foods that were enjoyed in the past. Again, it is a good idea to keep a journal or notebook to communicate this information with other caregivers.

- Can your loved one eat independently?

- Does your loved one have a visual impairment that may affect the ability to see a meal or drink? Left neglect might cause a person to ignore food on the left side of their plate. You would want to accommodate these impairments by setting the table accordingly.

- Due to normal age-related changes in eyesight, eating and dining may offer additional challenges—even if you're loved one suffered no visual impairment post-stroke.

- If your loved one is suffering from dysphagia after their stroke, precautions will need to be made to avoid aspiration of food into the airway. A special diet may need to be followed. Prior to leaving the hospital, you should meet with a dietician to be educated about your loved one's dietary needs.

- A soft food diet may need to be followed, or foods might need to be pureed or liquefied. Be sure the home has an appliance capable of performing this task.

### Eating—Communicating and Motivating

- Use short, simple sentences.

- Provide verbal cues and instructions as needed.

- Give your loved one your full attention.

- Be guiding, but not controlling.

### Eating—Routines and Preferences

- Factor into the overall daily schedule that it may take an hour or longer to finish each meal or snack.

- Keep mealtimes simple, and keep the routine that was familiar prior to your loved one's stroke. Encourage your loved one to eat in an upright position, especially if swallowing difficulties exist.

- If eating out was common, consider each restaurant's accessibility. Try to avoid rush hour, if extra time is needed. Make sure to get seating that fits a wheelchair or that optimizes independence. Even if dysphagia is an issue for your loved one, some restaurants will puree foods. Call ahead and inquire if your loved one's needs can be met at their facility.

**\*Note:** Remember, your loved one's sense of taste may change. Food that was eaten for years may no longer be enjoyable. Make note of any changes in your loved one's food preferences on the Personal History Form.

### Eating—Planning and Executing

This simple, everyday activity requires maneuvering objects, as well as other skills that many of us may take for granted. You and your loved one will need to develop techniques that work for your loved one. Again, document what is/isn't successful to communicate with other caregivers.

- It is completely appropriate to ask your loved one if assistance is desired.

- Offer to dish the food onto your loved one's plate if needed.

- Cut foods prior to serving if necessary. When cutting food, make sure the pieces are small enough for your loved one to chew and swallow easily.

If your loved one has visual deficits, create clear visual distinctions between the table, dishes, and the food.

- Use solid colors with no distracting patterns.

- When pouring a light-colored drink, such as milk, use a dark glass.

- When pouring a dark-colored drink, such as cola, use a white glass.

- Avoid clear glasses. They can disappear from view.

- Use white dishes when eating dark-colored food, and use dark dishes when eating light-colored food.

- If left neglect is present, keep everything within the right visual field. Put the items within their reach on the side of their strength.

- To make dishes easier to find on the table, use a tablecloth or placemats that are the opposite color of the dishes.

  **\*Note:** Fiesta ware colors (yellow/tangerine) contrast with most foods so they can be easily seen and will enhance visual perception.

- Use adaptive utensils if needed.

- Use a long straw with a no-spill cup or use a plastic mug with a large handle if needed.

## Other Meal Considerations

- If temperature discrepancy is limited, test the temperature of foods and beverages before serving.

- Make meals an enjoyable social event, so everyone looks forward to the experience.

- Clean up spills immediately.

- If your loved one wants to assist in making a meal, accommodate, and allow them to be safely involved. Give tasks that they will be successful at accomplishing.

## Meal Preparation Tips

Here are some tips to make meal preparation a little easier for your loved one:

- Labeling cabinets can improve independence by making it easier to locate items.

- Use simple, step-by-step written or verbal instructions.

- Consider writing out steps and checking off tasks as completed.

- Use proper equipment and modifications for food preparation. There is a variety of adaptive cooking tools available, from specialized cutting boards for one-handed individuals, built-up utensils, electric can openers, and timers for memory problems, to mats for stabilizing equipment. Some utensils can even gauge the temperature of the food.

- Provide supervision and/or assistance as needed to ensure your loved one's safety.

- When utilizing a stove top, use the back burners, and turn the handles inward toward the back of the stove. This technique can help avoid potential grabbing of the pots or pans, thus minimalizing a burn risk.

- If you are not there to supervise a meal due to work or other obligation, consider structuring and setting up the parts of the task so that your loved one can safely and independently complete them with success.

- If your loved one is able to manage basic food preparation, yet stove top cooking and/or cutting is problematic, consider putting individual meals in a microwaveable container with a label for cook time—or plan cold meals, such as sandwiches.

# Chapter 9

# Home Preparation

You and your loved one need to feel comfortable, capable, and safe in your home. As the Four Pillars of Engagement are the foundation for all activities, preparation of your home is crucial.

## General Organization and Environment

When organizing your loved one's environment, be sure to do it **_with_** them, not for them. Label drawers and cabinets, and make sure there is easy access to a phone. The following are general tips that caregivers and family members can use to prepare the home to accommodate your loved one's needs. Decide what works for you and your loved one.

## Home Safety Checklist: Bedroom

| Issue | Y/N | Options |
|-------|-----|---------|
| **Lighting**<br>Is lighting adequate? | | Add light-sensored night-light.<br><br>Place touch lamp on nightstand.<br><br>Place rope lighting along hallway leading to bathroom. |
| **Room Clutter**<br>Is there too much furniture, too many extra pillows, or too many "stacks of stuff"? | | Remove ALL extra furnishings and unnecessary "stacks of stuff."<br><br>Leave favorite items. |
| **Furniture Clutter**<br>Are dresser and nightstand cluttered? | | Remove ALL items from nightstand that are not functional and needed.<br><br>Leave the following items: lamp, phone, plastic drinking glass with top and straw, place for reading glasses and hearing aids.<br><br>Remove ALL unnecessary items from top of dresser to avoid confusion.<br><br>Remove unnecessary items and box for storage, donation, or disposal. |

| Home Safety Checklist: Bedroom | | |
|---|---|---|
| Issue | Y/N | Options |
| **Tripping Hazards**<br>Are there tripping hazards? | | Remove all throw and scatter rugs. Fix or replace loose floorboards. |
| Are there rugs or carpets that can be tripped on? | | Have professionals restretch loose carpeting to remove lumps and ridges if needed. |
| Are cords from lamps, TV, or radio out of the way? | | Move cords out of walking area. Bundle cords together and attach to baseboards or behind furniture. |
| Are pathways clear? | | Remove any loose items from floor or pathway from room. Organize and box for proper storage, donation, or disposal. |
| Is there enough room for walking aids? | | Make pathway wide enough to accommodate people, wheelchairs, and walking aids. |
| **Furniture**<br>Is furniture sturdy enough to provide support if needed? | | Antique bedside tables should be replaced with sturdy nightstands. |
| | | If possible, there should be a chair with sturdy arms and legs that is the same height as the bed. |
| Is bed a sensible height to get into and out of? | | Sensible height is if person's thighs are parallel to the floor and feet are flat on the floor when seated on edge of the bed. |
| | | Change out decorative bed frame for a practical bed frame if necessary. |

| Home Safety Checklist: Bedroom | | |
|---|---|---|
| Issue | Y/N | Options |
| **Bedding**<br>Is it sensible and practical?<br>Is it too heavy to be moved easily?<br><br>Is there an electric blanket or heating pad? | | Without removing your loved one's favorite blanket, lighten covers as much as possible.<br><br>Never use electric blankets or electric mattress pads.<br><br>Only use heating pads in chairs and never use for extended sleeping hours. |

| Home Safety Checklist: Closets | | |
|---|---|---|
| Issue | Y/N | Options |
| **Lighting**<br>Is lighting adequate?<br><br>Is light pull chain easily accessible? | | Install task lighting if needed.<br><br>If possible, change pull chain light fixture to light fixture with switch. |
| **Shelving**<br>Are shelves easy to reach?<br><br><br>Are shelves original from builder? | | Shelving should be located at a height that person using it can reach items without stretching.<br>Consider removing original shelving from builder and replacing with new, easier-access shelves. |
| **Shoes**<br>Can shoes be reached without bending over? | | If bending is an issue, consider installing an over-the-door shoe rack. |
| **Clothing**<br>Is closet full of clothing that is no longer being worn?<br><br><br><br><br><br>Are shelves stuffed with a hodgepodge of items that may tumble and fall? | | Never remove your loved one's favorite outfit.<br>Remove unworn or worn out clothing.<br>Leave choices that are easy to match.<br>Keep clothes that are easy to put on and take off.<br>Resolve shelving issue by removing unneeded items and organizing items to box and store, donate, or dispose of. |

## Home Safety Checklist: Bathroom

| Issue | Y/N | Options |
|---|---|---|
| **Lighting**<br>Is lighting adequate?<br><br>Is light switch easily accessible? | | Install task lighting if needed.<br><br>Change pull chain light to light with switch if possible. |
| **Color Contrast**<br>Is the bathroom all white or light colors? | | Change wall color so it contrasts with fixtures and counters. |
| **Toilet**<br>Is toilet at a height that allows your loved one to sit and stand comfortably? | | If possible, add a seat riser or a 3-in-1 commode over the toilet.<br>If possible, replace toilet with a taller model.<br><br>If possible, install grab bars on both sides at an angle that best suits person who needs them the most. |
| **Mirror**<br>Is mirror positioned for sitting and standing?<br><br><br>Does mirror cause fear or confusion? | | Mirrors may need to be covered  or removed for those with dementia as the person may no longer recognize themselves.<br><br>Mirrors can be removed or covered with a window shade that can be raised or lowered. |
| **Floor Mats and Rugs**<br>Is the bathroom floor all white or light colors? | | Use rug that is secured with double-sided tape or non-skid padding.<br><br>Don't use a dark rug—a person with dementia may mistake a dark rug for a hole in the floor. |

| Home Safety Checklist: Bathroom | | |
| --- | --- | --- |
| Issue | Y/N | Options |
| **Additional Seating**<br>Is the bathroom large enough for a chair? | | Use a chair in the bathroom to help your loved one while drying themselves after bath or to rest as needed. |
| **Temperature**<br>Is the bathroom warm enough? | | Some people may get cold easily and need the bathroom warmer than others. A portable heater could be used to warm the bathroom prior to use, but heater should be removed before using the bathroom. |
| **Tub/Shower**<br>Does tub/shower have decorative glass doors?<br><br>Are faucets clearly marked *Hot* and *Cold*?<br><br>Are shampoos, conditioners, and soaps in pump dispensers?<br><br>Is there a shower chair available? | | Remove glass doors and replace with a shower curtain.<br><br>Replace or remark *Hot* and *Cold* faucets.<br><br>Pump dispensers are easier to use than bottles that must be squeezed and/or turned upside down to dispense.<br><br>Showers can be exhausting. Using a shower chair to rest can help prevent someone from becoming too weak and falling during the shower. |
| **Grab Bars**<br>Are there grab bars to make getting into and out of tub or shower easier? | | Grab bars should be installed properly and securely into wall studs – not just into tile or fiberglass. Avoid use of suction cups as they can be unreliable. |

## Home Safety Checklist: Halls and Stairs

| Issue | Y/N | Options |
|---|---|---|
| **Lighting**<br>Is lighting adequate? | | Use a plug-in night-light. Install light switches on both ends of hallway. |
| **Obstacles**<br>Are there obstacles or clutter in hallway? | | Remove ALL clutter. Organize and box for proper storage, donation, or disposal—no matter what the item is. |
| Are there loose floorboards or rugs in hallway? | | Repair all loose floorboards. Remove all throw rugs. |
| Is there furniture in hallway? | | Remove all furniture. |
| Are there doors in hallway? | | Keep all doors closed at all times. |
| **Smoke/Carbon Monoxide Detectors**<br>Are carbon monoxide and smoke detectors installed? | | Install working units on all levels.<br><br>Replace batteries semiannually. |
| **Handrails**<br>Are there handrails in hallway and stairwell? | | Install handrails on both sides of hallway and stairwell or secure existing rails. |
| **Stairs**<br>Are steps easily seen? | | Use neon striping, paint, or duct tape to mark edges of stairs. |
| **Walkers**<br>Are walkers easily accessible and transportable? | | If possible, keep separate walkers at top and bottom of stairs. |

## Home Safety Checklist: Kitchen

| Issue | Y/N | Options |
|---|---|---|
| **Lighting**<br>Is lighting bright and adequate? | | Add task lighting as needed. Bright lights should be located in ceiling above table, countertops, sinks, stove, and in pantry. |
| **Smoke/Carbon Monoxide Detectors**<br>Are carbon monoxide and smoke detectors installed? | | Install detectors in kitchen.<br><br>Replace batteries semiannually. |
| **Fire Extinguisher**<br>Is there a fire extinguisher in the kitchen? | | Make sure fire extinguisher is usable and accessible. |
| **Appliances and their Cords**<br><br>Are there appliances in the kitchen that your loved one cannot or should not use?<br><br>Are there appliance cords that pose a danger? | | Remove appliances that should not or cannot be operated by your loved one on their own.<br><br>Make sure cords are not near sink or stove. |
| **Counter Clutter**<br>Are kitchen counters cluttered? | | Keep kitchen counters free of clutter that might cause confusion. |
| **Kitchen Floor**<br>Is floor free of tripping hazards? | | Remove all rugs, pet food bowls, cords, plants, or any other potential tripping hazards. |
| **Labels**<br>Are things visibly and legibly labeled? | | Create large-print labels for all switches and containers. |

## Home Safety Checklist: Kitchen

| Issue | Y/N | Options |
|---|---|---|
| **Cabinets** | | |
| Are doorknobs and cabinet handles easy to use? | | Label all cabinets and drawers, and replace difficult-to-use handles, pulls, or knobs. |
| Are the most-used items within easy reach? | | Rearrange cabinets if needed to make the most-used items easiest to reach. Get long-handled grabbers if needed. |
| Is assistance required to open jars and cans? | | Find adaptive tools that work best for your loved one. |
| **Stove** | | |
| Does it work properly? | | Make sure oven door and burner controls are easy to use and work properly. |
| Is it easy to use? | | Label burners and knobs/controls. |
| | | Clear all items on counters near stove. |
| Should it be used? | | If your loved one has a cognitive issue and shows signs of improper stove use, the caregiver must decide to unplug/ disconnect the stove. |
| | | Improper use can be things like: placing items on top of burners forgetting something is cooking forgetting that stove or oven is hot |
| **Microwave Oven** | | |
| Does your loved one know what it is and how to use it? | | Remove or unplug unit if needed. |

## Home Safety Checklist: Kitchen

| Issue | Y/N | Options |
|---|---|---|
| **Medication**<br><br>Are medications kept in the kitchen? | | Designate a cabinet for your loved one's medication.<br><br>If more than one person in home takes medication, use separate cabinets. |
| **Step Stools**<br><br>Should a step stool be used? | | Step stools can be a hazard and must not be used to reach items that are too high.<br><br>Find an alternative to a stool if items cannot be stored within person's reach. |
| **Refrigerator**<br><br>Is the food inside still good?<br><br><br>Is the food inside covered and stored properly?<br><br><br><br><br>Is a list of emergency contacts readily available on door? | | Designate someone to throw out old or rotten food. The person you are caring for may not know the difference.<br><br>All food in refrigerator and freezer should be tightly covered and stored properly with a label including what it is and date it was stored.<br><br>Do not store food on top of refrigerator –out of sight, out of mind!<br><br>Make sure emergency contact list and information is readily available in "File of Life" pouch on refrigerator door. |

## Home Safety Checklist: Living Area

| Issue | Y/N | Options |
|---|---|---|
| **Lighting**<br>Is lighting adequate? | | Room should be evenly lit throughout.<br><br>Use task lighting and touch lamps as needed. |
| **Flooring and Rugs**<br>Is the flooring free of clutter and tripping hazards? | | Remove and replace loose floorboards.<br><br>Area rugs are tripping hazards and should be removed.<br><br>If floor is carpeted, make sure it has been stretched properly, and ensure there are no lumps or ridges. |
| **Obstacles**<br>What are the obstacles in the room? | | Remove ALL clutter. Organize and box for proper storage, donation, or disposal—no matter what the item is. |
| Is there excess furniture? | | Remove unnecessary furniture. |
| Is there room to navigate? | | Allow 5½ feet in between each piece of furniture to accommodate use of a wheelchair. |
| Are there doors in the room? | | Keep all doors closed at all times. |
| **Tables**<br>Are there glass-topped tables? | | Remove all furniture with glass tops. |

## Home Safety Checklist: Living Area

| Issue | Y/N | Options |
|---|---|---|
| **Tables and Shelving** <br><br> Are tables and shelves full of clutter? | | Remove excess clutter from tables and shelves. Organize and box items for proper storage, disposal, or donation. |
| **Chairs and Seating** <br><br> Is the seating comfortable and easy to use? | | Use chairs with straight backs, armrests, and firm seats. <br><br> Make sure seating is a sensible height. Sensible height is if person's thighs are parallel to floor and feet are flat on the floor when seated on the edge of the chair. <br><br> If needed and possible, add firm cushion to existing pieces to add height. This will make it easier for your loved one to sit down and get up. |
| **Mirrors** <br><br> Does mirror cause fear or confusion? | | Mirrors may need to be covered or removed for those with dementia as the person may no longer recognize themselves. <br><br> Mirrors can be removed or covered with a window shade that can be raised or lowered. |
| **Cords** <br><br> Do they pose a tripping hazard? | | Use extension cords sparingly. Secure to baseboards to move them out of the way and prevent tripping. |

## Home Safety Checklist: Laundry

| Issue | Y/N | Options |
|---|---|---|
| **Lighting**<br>Is lighting adequate? | | Room should be bright. Add lighting as needed. |
| **Clutter and Organization**<br>Is room free of tripping hazards? | | If possible, find a place—other than on the floor—to store laundry basket.<br><br>Remove all unnecessary items and box for proper storage, donation, or disposal. |
| **Supplies**<br>Are laundry supplies organized and properly labeled?<br><br>Can laundry supplies be easily reached without stretching? | | Organize and label laundry supplies.<br><br><br>Ensure laundry supplies are within easy reach. |
| **Washer and Dryer**<br>Are washer and dryer easy and convenient to use?<br><br>Are dryer lint trap and vent hose cleaned regularly? | | Washer and dryer should be located side by side so that wet clothes do not have to be moved from room to room.<br>To prevent fires, clean lint trap and vent hose regularly. |
| **Ventilation**<br>Is the room well ventilated? | | Keep windows and/or doors open when in room for proper ventilation. |

## Home Safety Checklist: Basement

| Issue | Y/N | Options |
|---|---|---|
| **Stairs** Are there handrails on both sides of the steps? | | Install railings as needed. |
| Do railings or steps have loose or uneven wood or potential for splinters? | | Repair or replace wood that is loose or splintered. |
| Are items stacked on the steps? | | Remove unnecessary items and box for storage, donation, or disposal. |
| **Lighting** Is lighting adequate? | | Basement should be bright. Add lighting as needed. |
| Are light switches located at top and bottom of stairs? | | Install additional switches as needed. |
| **Clutter and Organization** Is room free of trip hazards? | | Remove unnecessary items and box for storage, donation, or disposal. |
| | | If possible, find a place—other than on the floor—to store laundry basket. |
| **Shelving** Is shelving sturdy enough to hold items placed on it? | | Remove unnecessary items and box for storage, donation, or disposal. |
| Are items on shelves neatly stacked so they will not fall off? | | Shelving should be located at a height that person using it can reach items without stretching. |
| **Frequently Used Items** Are frequently used items within easy reach? | | Organize items so that most-used items are easiest to reach. |

## Home Safety Checklist: Garage

| Issue | Y/N | Options |
|---|---|---|
| **Stairs** | | |
| Are there handrails on both sides of the steps? | | Install railings as needed. |
| Do railings or steps have loose or uneven wood or potential for splinters? | | Repair or replace wood that is loose, uneven, or splintered. |
| Are items stacked on the steps? | | Remove unnecessary items and box for storage, donation, or disposal. |
| **Lighting** | | |
| Is lighting adequate? | | Garage should be bright. Add lighting as needed. |
| Are light switches located at top and bottom of stairs? | | Install additional switches as needed. |
| **Tools and Equipment** | | |
| Are sharp tools away from walkways and hung or stored properly? | | Hang or store sharp tools properly for safety and to prevent tripping hazards. |
| Is machinery or equipment blocking walkway? | | Remove unnecessary items, and box for storage, donation, or disposal. |
| Are frequently used tools and equipment easily accessible? | | Organize space so that most-used items are easily accessible. |
| **Clutter and Organization** | | |
| Is room free of tripping hazards? | | Remove unnecessary items and box for storage, donation, or disposal. |

| Home Safety Checklist: Garage | | |
|---|---|---|
| Issue | Y/N | Options |
| **Frequently Used Items**<br><br>Are frequently used items easily accessible? | | If items are used inside the home, consider storing those items inside.<br><br>Remove unnecessary items, and box for storage, donation, or disposal. |
| **Garage Door**<br><br>Does garage door have an automatic opener? | | Automatic garage door openers make it easier to get in and out of the garage.<br><br>Check batteries in opener and in the main box semiannually. |

## Home Safety Checklist: Foyer

| Issue | Y/N | Options |
|-------|-----|---------|
| **Lighting**<br>Is lighting sufficient inside foyer and outside on porch? | | Add lighting as needed. |
| **Doorbell**<br>Can doorbell be heard all throughout home? | | Repair or replace doorbell so that it can be heard anywhere in the home. |
| **Door, Window, and Peephole**<br>Can you see who is standing on the front porch or stoop? | | Clear window or install peephole to be able to identify people before opening the door. |
| **Closet**<br>Is coat closet easy to use and not too cluttered?<br><br>Is there room to store hats, scarves, gloves, and boots? | | Remove unnecessary items and box for storage, donation, or disposal.<br><br>If there is no closet, install sturdy hooks for coats, hats, scarves, and gloves. |
| **Doormat**<br>Is there a doormat and is it appropriate? | | Use an absorbent mat with a non-skid backing.<br><br>Don't use a dark mat – a darker mat could be mistaken for a hole in the floor. |
| **Door**<br>Can door be easily locked?<br><br><br>Is there a dead bolt lock on the door? | | If a person is in early stages of dementia, doors should be secured to prevent wandering.<br><br>Install latches high on door so they cannot be easily reached. |

| Home Safety Checklist: Porch, Yard, Driveway | | |
|---|:---:|---|
| Issue | Y/N | Options |
| **Lighting** | | |
| Do exterior porch and garage lights illuminate entire areas? | | Add lighting or replace bulbs with the highest wattage the fixture allows. |
| Is yard lighting equipped with motion detectors? | | If possible, install motion detector lights for safety and security. |
| **Steps and Rails** | | |
| Are there sturdy rails to use for climbing up and down stairs? | | Repair or replace rails as needed to ensure proper sturdiness and safety. |
| Are rails smooth and free of splinters? | | Repair or replace rails to prevent injury from cracks or splinters. |
| Are there any loose or wobbly steps? | | Repair or replace any loose or wobbly steps to prevent trip/fall hazard. |
| Are steps slippery in wet conditions? | | Add non-slip material to stair treads to prevent them from becoming slippery when wet. |
| **Sidewalks and Driveway** | | |
| Do sidewalks and driveway have cracks or loose cement that could be trip hazards? | | Repair any cracks or loose cement that could be potential trip hazards. Be aware of tree roots that may affect paved surfaces. |
| **Mailbox** | | |
| Is there a clear path to the mailbox? | | Make arrangements with the Post Office to have mail delivered to door for a person who is elderly or disabled. |

## Lighting, Glare, and Color Contrast

Depending on your loved one's vision, the severity of a brain injury or cognitive deficit, or individual preferences, you may find it necessary to modify existing lighting, glare, and contrast in the home. People will not always admit that they have an issue with their vision, but if they do, it will affect their ability to engage in an activity. Here are some tips to help:

### Lighting

The following lighting changes could be key in your loved one's safety and ability to perform tasks independently.

- Fluorescent lighting can contribute to an increase in glare. Try different types of lightbulbs to see which is most comfortable for your loved one.

- Keep all rooms evenly lit and the lighting level consistent throughout the home, so shadows and dangerous bright spots are eliminated.

- Make sure light switches, pull cords, and lamps are easily accessible for your loved one, particularly if he or she is in a wheelchair.

- If possible, purchase touch lamps or those that can be turned on or off by sound.

- Be certain that all stairwells are well lit and have handrails.

- Depending on the individual, additional task lighting may be necessary in certain areas of the home.

- Additional lighting for closets and smaller areas may be helpful. Battery-operated push lights are a good option.

## Glare

Glare can be caused by sunlight or light from a lamp. When the light hits a shiny surface, such as a magazine page or even a wall painted with high-gloss paint, the resulting glare can make it difficult for someone with low vision to see.

Sunglasses can be beneficial for someone who is light sensitive. Offer your loved one the opportunity to try different lens colors to see which works best.

- Sunlight can fill the room with light without producing glare. Adjust sunlight coming through windows by using mini blinds and altering their position throughout the day. If mini blinds are not available, use sheer curtains to diffuse the light.

- Be aware when placing mirrors in a room. Mirrors placed across from larger windows can significantly increase the amount of light in a room. This could be beneficial for someone who prefers the additional light.

- Cover bare lightbulbs with shades.

- Position chairs and tables so that when your loved one is sitting on a chair or at a table, they are not looking directly at the light coming from a window.

- Cover or remove shiny/reflective surfaces, such as floors and tabletops.

## Color Contrasts

Using contrast is a good strategy if your loved one has a visual impairment. The more contrast, the easier it is to find and use objects or activity items around the house.

- Put light-colored objects against a dark background.

- Avoid upholstery with patterns for seated activities. Stripes, plaids, and checks can be visually confusing.

- Opt for solid-colored tables and countertops in a neutral tone.

Countertops with busy patterns can make it difficult to locate items and can be more difficult to keep clean.

- In a room with mostly dark tones, place light-colored pillows or chairs in strategic places to help your loved one find things and get around easily.

- If your loved one must, or is capable of maneuvering stairs, put contrasting stripes on the edges of each stair to make each stair visible and to prevent the stairs from disappearing from view.

# Chapter 10

# Put Your Mask on First

There will be many challenges to you personally in this caregiving journey that can and will wear you down. As a caregiver, first and foremost, you must take care of yourself in order to be able to assist your loved one. That might be easier said than done, but please make every effort to do so. The following are some general tips for you, the family caregiver:

**About You**

- Put yourself first (this is not being selfish) —if you are not in good physical or mental health you cannot help anyone.
- Arrange some time for yourself.
- Keep a strong support system.
- Do not be afraid to ask for help.
- Keep contact with friends.
- Define priorities; do not try to be all things to all people.

## Stress

- Recognize your own stress and take steps to minimize. Stress can be exhibited in multiple ways:
  - Anger
  - Helplessness
  - Embarrassment
  - Grief
  - Depression
  - Isolation
  - Physical illness

## Burnout

Burnout for caregivers results from physical and emotional exhaustion.

It is important to realize a family member, spouse, or hired caregiver experiences the same emotions as staff in health care facilities, but may not have the needed support system. Suggestions to avoid burnout:

- Know what makes you angry or impatient. Make a list.

- Look for the reason behind behavior.
- Use relaxation techniques, e.g., deep breathing, imagery, and music.
- Ask for help, and accept help when it is offered!

Caregiving is a challenging road with constant twists and turns, from the change in your role/relationship with your loved one, to dealing with the strains of a 24/7 job of caring for that loved one. As much as you may feel like you are alone, please know that you are not. Millions of family caregivers are dealing with the same issues that you are. Do not be embarrassed to share details about what you are experiencing, and do not be afraid to ask for help. There are individuals, organizations, and support groups throughout the country that are available to you. There is also R.O.S. —we were built on the simple mission of our founder's need to help his mother and father during a 25-year battle with Parkinson's and dementia. We understand what you are going through, and we are here to help.

# Personal History Form

*This is* _____ *'s Personal History*

Name: _____

Maiden Name: _____

Preferred Name: _____

Date of Birth: _____

Place of Birth: _____

Name and relationship of people completing this Personal
History Form: _____

_____

_____

_____

_____

Describe the person's personality prior to the stroke.

_____

_____

_____

_____

_____

_____

_____

What makes the person feel valued? Talents, occupation, accomplishments, family, etc. _____

_____

_____

_____

What are the daily living aids that must always be handy?

_____

_____

_____

What are some favorite items they must always have in sight or close by? _____

_____

_____

What is their exact morning routine? _____

_____

_____

_____

What is their exact evening routine? _____

_____

_____

_____

What type of clothing do they prefer? Do they like to choose their own clothes for the day, or do they prefer to have their clothes laid out by someone else?

_____

_____

_____

_____

_____

What is their favorite beverage?

_____

What is their favorite food?

_____

_____

What will get them motivated? (Church, friends coming over, going out, etc.)

_____

_____

_____

_____

_____

_____

_____

List significant interests in their life, such as hobbies, recreational activities, job related skills/experiences, military experience, etc.

- Age 8 to 20:

_____

_____

_____

- Age 20 to 40:

_____

_____

_____

- Age 40+:

_____

_____

_____

What is their religious background?  (Affiliation, prayer time, symbols, traditions, church/synagogue name, etc. Did they lead any services or sing in the choir?)

_____

_____

_____

_____

What type of music do they enjoy listening to, playing, or singing?  Do they have any musical talents?

_____

_____

_____

What is their favorite TV program?  Movie?

_____

_____

_____

If reading has been a hobby, what authors, topics, or genres do they prefer?  Would they listen to audiobooks or books on tape?

_____

_____

_____

_____

Marital status - If married more than once, provide specifics. Include names of spouses, dates of marriage, and other relevant information.

_____

_____

_____

_____

List distinct characteristics about their spouse(s), such as occupations, personality traits, or daily routine.

_____

_____

_____

_____

_____

Do they have children? Be sure to include children both living and deceased. Include names, birth dates, and any other relevant information.

_____

_____

_____

_____

_____

Do they have siblings? Be sure to include siblings both living and deceased. Include names, birth dates, and any other relevant information.

_____

_____

_____

_____

137

Who do they ask for the most?  What is their relationship with this person(s)?  Describe how that person typically spends their day.

_____

_____

_____

_____

What causes them stress? How is stress exhibited? Are there particular triggers like loud noises or being ignored?

_____

_____

_____

_____

What calms them down when they are stressed or agitated?

_____

_____

_____

_____

How long has it been since the stroke occurred?

_____

_____

Describe how the symptoms are affecting your loved one.

_____

_____

_____

_____

_____

Have they accepted the changes in life since the stroke?

_____

_____

_____

What activities do they feel can no longer be participated in as a result of the stroke? And why?

_____

_____

_____

_____

What specific activities did they enjoy prior to the stroke?

_____

_____

_____

_____

Are they participating less frequently with family and friends? Can you identify why?

_____

_____

_____

_____

_____

_____

What age do you think the person thinks they are?

_____

Do they ask for their spouse but do not recognize them?

_____

Do they look for their children but do not recognize them?

_____

Do they look for their mom? _____

Do they perceive themselves as younger? Please describe.

_____

_____

Describe the "home" they remember. _____

_____

_____

_____

Can they tell the difference between someone on TV and a real person?

_____

_____


Other information that would help to bring joy to your loved one.

_____

_____

_____

_____

_____

_____

_____

_____

_____

_____

_____

_____

_____

_____

_____

_____

_____

_____

_____

_____

_____

_____

_____

_____

_____

_____

_____

_____

_____

_____

_____

_____

_____

_____

_____

* **Note:** This form includes questions being asked in case your loved one has dementia symptoms that are caused by their stroke.

| P = past interest, **C** = currently engages in this activity, **NEW** = Has expressed interest in learning | | | | |
|---|---|---|---|---|
| **NAME:** | | | | |
| Interest | N/A | P | C | New |
| **Arts and Crafts** | | | | |
| Knitting | | | | |
| Sewing | | | | |
| Crocheting | | | | |
| Embroidering | | | | |
| Scrapbooking | | | | |
| Painting type: | | | | |
| Coloring | | | | |
| Woodworking | | | | |
| Other | | | | |
| **Table Games** | | | | |
| Cards type: | | | | |
| Bingo | | | | |
| Dominoes | | | | |
| Board Games | | | | |
| Pokeno | | | | |
| Jigsaw Puzzles | | | | |
| Other: | | | | |
| **Spiritual** | | | | |
| Attend Church/Synagogue/Temple/Mosque | | | | |
| Rosary Service | | | | |
| Bible trivia | | | | |
| Bible study | | | | |
| Reading Bible/Torah/Koran/Watchtower | | | | |
| Other: | | | | |

| P = past interest, **C** = currently engages in this activity, **NEW** = Has expressed interest in learning | | | | |
|---|---|---|---|---|
| **NAME:** | | | | |
| Interest | N/A | P | C | New |
| **Television / Movies** | | | | |
| Favorite channel: | | | | |
| Movie types: | | | | |
| Soap Operas: | | | | |
| Game Shows: | | | | |
| Talk Shows: | | | | |
| Comedies: | | | | |
| Dramas: | | | | |
| News: | | | | |
| Westerns: | | | | |
| Cartoons: | | | | |
| Adult Films: | | | | |
| Other: | | | | |
| **Reading / Writing** | | | | |
| Book Club | | | | |
| Type of Books: | | | | |
| Large Print | | | | |
| Talking Books | | | | |
| Magazines: | | | | |
| Legacy Kits/Autobiography | | | | |
| Newspaper: | | | | |
| Word Search | | | | |
| Crossword Puzzles | | | | |
| Letter Writing | | | | |
| Other: | | | | |

| P = past interest, **C** = currently engages in this activity, **NEW** = Has expressed interest in learning | | | | |
|---|---|---|---|---|
| **NAME:** | | | | |
| Interest | N/A | P | C | New |
| **Sports   Play or Watch** | | | | |
| Exercise: | | | | |
| Baseball Team: | | | | |
| Football Team: | | | | |
| Soccer Team: | | | | |
| Golf Player: | | | | |
| Basketball Team: | | | | |
| NASCAR Driver: | | | | |
| Tennis Player: | | | | |
| Other: | | | | |
| **Musical Interests** | | | | |
| Singing | | | | |
| Listening to Radio/CD Type: | | | | |
| Live Music | | | | |
| Play Instrument: | | | | |
| Movies / Videos | | | | |
| **Outdoor Activities** | | | | |
| Gardening | | | | |
| Shopping / Outings | | | | |
| Traveling | | | | |
| Hunting | | | | |
| Fishing | | | | |
| Smoking | | | | |
| Other: | | | | |

| P = past interest, **C** = currently engages in this activity, **NEW** = Has expressed interest in learning | | | | |
|---|:---:|:---:|:---:|:---:|
| **NAME:** | | | | |
| Interest | N/A | P | C | New |
| **Technology** | | | | |
| Computers / Internet | | | | |
| Hand-held Video Games: | | | | |
| TV Video Games: | | | | |
| Other: | | | | |
| **Volunteering** | | | | |
| Distributing Mail: | | | | |
| Newsletters: | | | | |
| Church Groups: | | | | |
| Service Projects: | | | | |
| Other: | | | | |
| **Social Activities** | | | | |
| Men's Groups / Ladies' Groups / Young Person's Groups: | | | | |
| Happy Hour | | | | |
| Coffee Club | | | | |
| Intergenerational Visits | | | | |
| Discussion Groups | | | | |
| History Groups | | | | |
| **Other** | | | | |
| Cooking: | | | | |
| Animals: | | | | |
| Political Interest: | | | | |
| Manicures | | | | |
| Other: | | | | |

# About the Authors

### Scott Silknitter

Scott Silknitter is the founder of R.O.S. Therapy Systems. He designed and created the R.O.S. Play Therapy™ System, the *How Much Do You Know About* Series of themed activity books, and the R.O.S. *BIG Book*. Starting with a simple backyard project to help Mom and Dad, Scott has dedicated his life to improving the quality of life for all seniors through meaningful education, entertainment, and activities.

### Suzanne John, RN

Suzanne John is a retired Registered Nurse. She possesses over 12 years of clinical nursing experience in areas, such as Cardiothoracic Surgical nursing, Medical and Cardiac Intensive Care nursing, working with ventilator-dependent patients and their families in a long-term care facility, Supervising RN in a skilled nursing facility, and as a RN providing outpatient cardiac rehab care to patients post open-heart surgery or after a "heart attack." Suzanne believes, "a nurse should be intelligent in her knowledge of the human body and medicine to practice safe care, but a nurse's success is obtained in her ability to interact and relate to her patient's condition and establish a trusting and respectful relationship." Suzanne currently teaches students studying to earn a caregiver certificate how to perform Activities of Daily Living.

## Alisa Tagg, BA, ACC/EDU, AC-BC, CDP

Alisa Tagg is a Certified Activity Consultant with a specialization in Education and a Certified Dementia Practitioner. With over 25 years of experience, Alisa is an authorized certification instructor for the Modular Education Program for Activity Professionals. Alisa currently serves on the National Association of Activity Professionals as the president.

# References

1. *The Handbook of Theories on Aging* (Bengtson et al., 2009)
2. *Activity Keeps Me Going, Volume 1*, (Peckham et al., 2011)
3. *Essentials for the Activity Professional in Long-Term Care* (Lanza, 1997)
4. *Abnormal Psychology*, Butcher
5. www.dhspecialservices.com
6. National Certification Council for Dementia Practitioners www.NCCDP.org
7. "Managing Difficult Dementia Behaviors: An A-B-C Approach" By Carrie Steckl
8. Iowa Geriatric Education Center website, Marianne Smith, PhD, ARNP, BC Assistant Professor University of Iowa College of Nursing
9. *Excerpts taken from "Behavior...Whose Problem is it?" Hommel, 2012
10. *Merriam-Webster's Dictionary*
11. "The Latent Kin Matrix" (Riley, 1983)
12. *Care Planning Cookbook* (Nolta et al.2007)
13. "Long-Term Care" (Blasko et al. 2011)
14. Success Oriented Programs for the Dementia Client (Worsley et al 2005)
15. Heerema, Esther. "Eight Reasons Why Meaningful Activities Are Important for People with Dementia." www.about.com
16. *Activities 101 for the Family Caregiver* (Appler-Worsley, Bradshaw, Silknitter)
17. American Foundation for the Blind
18. www.aging.com
19. www.WebMD.com
20. www.caregiver.org
21. American Stroke Association
22. www.dysphagiadiet.com
23. *Textbook of Medical-Surgical Nursing*, Brunner/Suddarth, 5th edition

For additional assistance, please contact us at:
www.ROSTherapySystems.com
888-352-9788

Made in the USA
Columbia, SC
29 May 2023

17130431R00087